Back to Nature with Linda

A Helpful Guide to the Uses and Healing Powers of Essential Oils

Linda Strom Medvitz

facebook.com/linda.strommedvitz

www.youngliving.org/lindasmedvitz

soslindas@gmail.com

Limits of Liability and Disclaimer of Warranty

The author/publisher shall not be liable for your misuse of this material. This book is strictly for informational and educational purposes.

Warning – Disclaimer

The purpose of this book is to educate and entertain. It is distributed with the understanding that the publisher is not engaged in the dispensation of legal, psychological or any other professional advice. The content of each entry is the expression and opinion of its author and does not necessarily reflect the beliefs, practices or viewpoints of the publisher, its parent company or its affiliates. The publisher's choice to include any material within is not intended to express or imply any warranties or guarantees of any kind. The author and/or publisher do not guarantee that anyone following these techniques, suggestions, tips, ideas, or strategies will become successful. The author and/or publisher shall have neither liability nor responsibility to anyone with respect to any loss or damage caused, or alleged to be caused, directly or indirectly by the information contained in this book.

DISCLAIMER: This information is not presented by a medical practitioner and is for educational and informational purposes only. The content is not intended to be a substitute for professional medical advice, diagnosis, or treatment. Always seek the advice of your physician or other qualified health care provider with any questions you may have regarding a medical condition. Never disregard professional medical advice or delay in seeking it because of something you have read.

ISBN-13: 978-1979564762

ISBN-10: 1979564760

"How we live, work and play have changed in exciting ways. Our world activities have speeded up so much that it is hard to keep balance at times. Young Living Oils are a great help to keep that balance."

~ **Linda Strom Medvitz**

What People Are Saying About Linda and Young Living Oils

From Tom Medvitz: *I encourage people to use the acknowledged "pharmacology of the ancients" to cure the ills of the present. Young Living Oils provide just that—a way to use the secret tools and techniques of the past to deal with the stressors and illnesses of today.*

From Saida Smith: *Working with Linda and Young Living Oils has been a wonderful experience. Linda has helped me to teach women, mothers and anyone interested in a more natural, holistic life how and why to use pure essential oils to heal and balance their lives.*

From Christopher Mason: *Many years ago a massage therapist used essential oils during my session and preformed what is called the "raindrop technique" on me. Ever since then I have been hooked on oils and enjoy them for their countless health benefits. I signed up as a distributor so that I could get the oils at wholesale and have had a few people do the same thing. Thank you, Linda and others, for introducing me to this wonderful resource!*

From Donna Bair: *I have used Young Living Oils for many years. I include the oils in my practice as a Hospice RN, as they help to bring calm and peace during a difficult time in the lives of patients and families. Young Living Oils are an important part of caring for my family and friends in our hectic daily life. Now I am learning to incorporate the Young Living Oils and music to enhance my healing practice. Working with Linda has expanded my ideas of how the oils can be used and who can use them. It's a wonderful ride with Linda and Young Living Oils!*

From Gayle Brown of Running Quail Ranch: *We love Young Living Oils and their fabulous supplements. We use them with all the animals and their owners. They work wonders on both people and pets!*

About Linda Strom Medvitz

To say Linda Strom Medvitz is a go-getter is putting it mildly.

It all started by having a strong role model, her mother. Linda comes from strong stock. Born in San Diego, Linda's mother, Marjorie L. Reed, conquered a lot of "firsts."

"She was the first woman to do many things," said Linda. "My dad wanted Mom to stay home, take care of four kids and cook and clean. My mother was smart and ambitious. She wanted to work, and she got jobs with the school system as a secretary. She worked, even when he didn't want her to. They divorced when I was 12."

Her mother worked and succeeded with money, becoming a millionaire several times over. "She was my inspiration all along, because she raised four kids herself," said Linda.

And the apple didn't fall far from the tree. Mom, being the role model that she was, got involved with the education system early on. As Linda said, her mom first worked in the San Diego City School System as a secretary. From there she worked up to administrative leadership. She then obtained a real estate license, and the rest is history. But the itch to start her own business was always with her. Growing up with her mother, Linda learned to be capable and confident. "My mom had been independent, so why couldn't I be independent?"

Linda married and family came soon after as she had two daughters. Things were rough nearly from the start, though, and the marriage didn't work out. Linda and her girls ended up back at her mom's house. Two strong-willed women in one house led to tension, with Linda searching for her next step.

It came while her mother was in Europe and Linda had an opportunity to buy a condo. (This was in the 1970s when investing in condos was all the rage.) It took some financial finagling because women weren't allowed to get their own credit cards, let alone purchase property then, but Linda bought the condo while her mother was away. "When she returned, she was livid. But I was independent because that's how I was raised," Linda said.

"I am my mother's daughter. She was a good example."

When Linda met her second husband in 1975, she had two condos, two kids, and worked two jobs. "It wasn't popular for women to do what I did, but that's just the type of person I've been," said Linda.

She and her husband decided to go into condominium management and served on the Board of Directors in a 350-unit condominium complex. "We were self-managed and I became President of the Board. The board didn't know what they were doing, so we shaped it up and hired a management company and went from there," Linda said. She and her husband then bought a condominium in a complex of 108 units in Santee, and became members of that Board of Directors. Linda was then hired by the management company to manage other condominium associations.

Linda and her husband decided to start their own Condominium Management Company in 1983. "We had our condominium business for 20 years. We had 15 employees who we are still in contact with. They were like family," she said. "I've been one to not be afraid to jump out, move forward and do something. Don't tell me I can't do it, because I will."

Linda faced a few more times in her life when she had to dig deep to find her own strength. Here's the way she tells one of those stories:

"I had a spot in my life, it's been almost three years now, where I had an issue with my heart. I kept going to the doctors and they kept giving me stuff and sending me home. They couldn't find the issue. After six months they finally did: three of my veins in my heart were blocked. They were 80% Occluded. The reason they didn't find it in X-rays is because they were blocked evenly—usually it's 20%, 30%, or 40%. When you're at 30%, you could have heart attacks or other problems. I was sent into surgery and I had three stents installed.

"The surgeon saved my life. Because of that, they gave me seven different medications to take. I had to take medicine for cholesterol, which I didn't have prior to the operation. I mean, all this stuff I had to take knocked me on my butt. I was almost bedridden. I couldn't drive, I couldn't function for six months.

"Well, I had never prayed much but I started praying. What came up was Young Living Oils. I decided I was going to get off all the medications. The cardiologist thought I would die if I quit all the stuff that he had prescribed, but I knew I couldn't continue living like that. In the end we parted with him telling me, 'I will pray for you.'

"Now I'm only on one of those pharmaceuticals, a thyroid pill. I got off of all of them. I'm not sick. I'm healthy and I'm driving.

"Once I got off the medications and was no longer miserable and sick, what was I going to do? The answer seemed obvious. I chose to share Young Living Oils. I decided to work with the oils that heal. I had to be sick and stuck in bed, being told I was dying, to realize that there was something else out there. Young Living Oils have always inspired me, but now I'm making them my life's work."

Linda and her husband had another close call in 2003, when fire swept through their area and they lost everything. Even so, she doesn't resent the fire. "Fire is natural, just like our oils are natural. Fire had to happen to cleanse the land to recreate new growth," she said. They started over with nothing, not even insurance money, as a weird turn of events led it to lapse a few weeks prior to the fires.

"I had to go back to work for obvious reasons, and we had to rebuild. Life was a challenge. We started over with nothing but the clothes on our backs," she said.

"But we got to experience humanity as an outpouring of love and giving for the fire victims. The home we are living in now is only 620 square feet and it was built by Salvation Army volunteers," said Linda. "Then it was back to work for me—retirement was over."

The challenge wasn't new for Linda, and she once again dug deep and got it done.

She said, "I think going through these harrowing experiences made me realize that I'm not done yet. I'm not."

Table of Contents

How Essential Oils Are Made

"Work, love and play are the great balance wheels of man's being."
~ Orison Swett Marden

ESSENTIAL OILS are extracts from certain plants, trees, and fruits using a technique called distillation. Since plants contain only a small amount of extract, several pounds of plants are needed to provide a small bottle of an essential oil to consumers. The essential oils are then refined and distilled and packaged in containers that help maintain the scent and fragrance for a good amount of time. The following is a list of treatments and extraction procedures that produce the essential oils for our use in aromatherapy or creams.

Steam Distillation

Steam distillation is the most popular and the oldest distillation process available. Old time, traditional aromatherapy professionals believe this method is the best way to produce the most quality extracts. This system takes dried or fresh plants and places them into a steam chamber. The steam is put under pressure and then circulated in and out of the plant material. The heat from the pressurized steam causes the plant's cellular structure to open, and the essential oils pour into a holding container. This is a delicate method since the heat must be well balanced to open the plant but not too hot causing destruction of the delicate oil.

After the steam and oil are distilled into a container, the steam returns to a liquid while the oil creates a film at the top of the solution. Both the liquid and the oil are therapeutic by-products of the process. The oils can be packaged as pure essential oil extract. The water still holds a lot of the oil properties, so it is used by cosmetic companies in toners or skin creams.

Cold Pressing

Extracts from fruits such as bergamot, grapefruit, lemon or limes use different forms of processing. The essential oils are mainly in the fruit's peel, so it needs to be penetrated. The fruit's peel is rolled over a large array of sharp objects that cause the peel to burst, and the oils are extracted. Then the fruit is squeezed and the juice contained. The essential oils rise to the top of the juices as a film like in steam distillation. They are separated by centrifugation into containers that are packaged for consumers.

Effleurage

This method of extraction is used for flowers or plants that are very delicate. Some plants are too delicate to withstand the heat from steam distillation. Effleurage uses animal fat to absorb the essential oils from the delicate flowers. As the petals are depleted of their oils, more are placed on the animal fats until it is completely saturated with the extract. After the fat is saturated, the fat is treated with alcohol, which solvates the essential oils. Once the mixture is contained, the alcohol will evaporate, leaving behind the essential oil product.

Solvent Extraction

Solvent extraction is the most efficient and affordable way to separate the extract from the plant. In this method, a solvent is used to saturate the plant and absorb the oils. After saturation, it is then treated with alcohol. Like effleurage, the alcohol eventually evaporates and it leaves only the essential oils for packaging. This method is especially useful for more expensive extracts where each plant needs to be squeezed for as much extract as possible. Although this method is the most cost efficient, it can leave solvent in the product, which can cause side effects.

How to Use Essential Oils Properly

"The joy of life comes from our encounters with new experiences, and hence there is no greater joy than to have an endlessly changing horizon, for each day to have a new and different sun."
~ Christopher McCandless

DEPENDING ON your needs, first you will want to carefully choose which essential oil is best for you. Are you looking for an essential oil that might help with your mood or to decrease stress? There are many mood-enhancing essential oils that can be used in aromatherapy for mental fatigue, stress, and anxiety. Are you hoping to use essential oils to help with skin breakouts, rashes, or bug bites? There are several possible essential oils that can be diluted and applied topically to help with these issues. Consult a professional or an essential guidebook to determine what essential oil would best benefit you and your situation.

Consult a professional or an essential guidebook to determine what essential oil would best benefit you and your situation.

It is important to use the proper essential oil in the proper way or you may find yourself frustrated that they don't work.

Spread the essential oil cream on a small area of your skin and observe for twenty-four hours.

After you choose an essential oil it is important to test it prior to using it. Essential oils should never be applied without testing a small area of the skin. The oils should also never be used without first diluting the extract. Essential oils are potent, so using them on the skin without diluting can cause a rash or burn. Conversely, dilute a small drop in a few milliliters of vegetable oil. Spread the essential oil cream on a small area of your skin and observe for twenty-four hours. If your skin becomes irritated or red, then you may be allergic to that specific oil. Use this method even before burning essential oils for aromatherapy.

Consult a professional for information on which use is most effective for a particular essential oil.

After checking for allergies, it is time to use the essential oils. There are several different methods that you can use. Consult a professional for information on which use is most effective for a particular essential oil. Below is a list of ways to inhale or apply the essential oils for the different therapeutic effects. It is important to use each essential oil the way it is intended for the best benefits.

Proper Ways to Inhale Essential Oils

Diffuser

A diffuser will allow you to inhale the essential oils. Put a few drops of essential oils into the diffuser with water. Some essential oils can be used just with the heat, so make sure to read the directions. A diffuser will evaporate the essential oils into the air, and most come with a timer so that they can be used while sleeping.

Dry Evaporation

Dry evaporation is a more simple way to inhale the essential oils. You can place a few drops on a cotton swap or tissue and allow it to evaporate into the air. If you need a quick, strong scent, inhale the fragrance directly from the cotton swap. For a less potent effect, allow the essential oils to evaporate on the tissue or cotton swap and leave it in the general vicinity of where you will remain for about an hour.

Steam

Steam is a simple way to inhale the essential oil aroma. Place a few drops into a steaming bowl of water. The oils will quickly vaporize into the air. Place a towel over your head and place your head close to the steam and inhale. The fresh fragrance of the essential oils will penetrate your senses and help you feel refreshed.

Proper Ways to Apply Essential Oils

Although essential oils are a mild, natural way to help fight off mental fatigue, stress, sore muscles, and other physical conditions, they are also very potent and need to be applied properly. After you have purchased the perfect essential oils for your condition, it is important to know how to apply them. If used without proper direction, they can have a negative effect which can frustrate you. They may even cause harm if not applied properly.

First, using undiluted essential oils directly on your skin can harm rather than help your condition. Used directly on the skin, essential oils can sometimes leave a rash or a burn. The essential oils are powerful solutions to many issues, but used improperly they can cause painful sores when directly applied to the skin. Diluting the essential oils in cream or non-greasy oil will keep it from strongly affecting your skin.

Essential oils are absorbed by your skin quickly, so use caution.

Like many creams or lotions, spreading essential oils directly on the skin can cause an overdose. Essential oils are absorbed by your skin quickly, so use caution. If the oil that you are applying isn't diluted, it can lead to an overdose that will cause a rash, irritation, or skin breakout. It is also important not to have overexposure to sun, especially if you've accidentally applied too much. Essential oils and sun exposure can lead to adverse effects.

Even though essential oils are naturally occurring extracts from plants and trees, they are also powerful therapeutic agents. It is important to keep them out of the reach of children. Spreading essential oils undiluted onto a child's skin can be dangerous and leave a very painful breakout rash. When applying essential oils be sure to keep it away from your eyes, nose, or ears.

Before fully using essential oils, remember to make sure to test them on a very small part of your skin. This includes essential oils that you may use in aromatherapy. Apply a small dab to your arm and observe any reaction for twenty four hours. For essential oils that you will apply as a cream, dilute the oil into vegetable oil and apply to the skin. Observe for any reaction for twenty-four hours to make sure they are safe for topical use.

Essential Oils for Aromatherapy

"Joy is what happens to us when we allow ourselves to recognize how good things really are."
~ Marianne Williamson

ESSENTIAL OILS can be used for many things, but are most often used in aromatherapy. This is when you take advantage of the scents of the oils, which can then heal your mind and body.

Aromatherapy with essential oils helps with many different ailments, including physical and mental ones. Here are some examples of what you can use essential oils and aromatherapy for:

- Mental health disorders like stress, anxiety, and depression
- Headaches and migraines
- Joint aches, arthritis, muscular conditions
- Inflammation and weak immune system
- To relax the nervous system
- Insomnia
- Acute or chronic pain
- Certain symptoms of pregnancy

With aromatherapy, you want to inhale the scented oil in order to get the full effect. Try some of these popular essential oils for aromatherapy purposes.

Peppermint

If you want to give aromatherapy with essential oils a try, go with something mild and minty like peppermint. This is a strong and effective essential oil that can help with anything from sore muscles to digestive issues. It is also really good for headaches and migraines, as well as congestion, cold, and flu symptoms. A good carrier oil for peppermint essential oil is grapeseed oil.

Eucalyptus

Eucalyptus is also a strong essential oil that you can try using for aromatherapy purposes. Eucalyptus can be a strong, earthy scent, but don't let that fool you; this oil is very soothing and can open your airways. It is also great for relieving muscle pain, helping with asthma and congestion, and even providing dental and skin care benefits. If you prefer, you can put some drops in your bath, which still allows the benefits, without the strong scent.

Lavender

Lavender is one of the most popular essential oils to use for aromatherapy, especially if you need help with insomnia, stress, anxiety, or depression. You will find the subtle floral scent to be very soothing and calming. Add it to your bath at night to relax enough to sleep or apply it with a carrier oil to your skin to help with burns or insect bites. It can also be used for muscle or joint pain.

Essential Oils for Allergies

"So divinely is the world organized that every one of us, in our place and time, is in balance with everything else."
~ Johann Wolfgang von Goethe

IF YOU suffer from allergies, you might be looking for a natural remedy. Essential oils are an exceptional way to help get rid of your allergy symptoms and start to experience relief. Here are some things to know about using essential oils for your allergies.

How Essential Oils Can Help

Before you learn about the best essential oil blends for allergies, it helps to know exactly how the oils can help with allergies. One of the main ways they can help is by boosting your immune system. Many of the listed essential oils not only boost your immune system so allergens don't affect you as much, but they can also help to fight inflammation, which is a major contributor to allergy symptoms. Using the oils regularly will help tremendously.

Peppermint

A good essential oil to start with when you want to ease your allergy symptoms is peppermint. With peppermint, it works really great when you are already experiencing your allergy symptoms. It can help with digestive problems and the aroma is really good at helping you to breathe easier, which is often a concern among allergy sufferers. Peppermint can help with skin irritation, inflammation, and most types of allergic reactions. You can either apply diluted peppermint oil around your nostrils or use it in your bath. It can also be used with aromatherapy.

Eucalyptus

Another good essential oil to try is eucalyptus, which is great for allergies and respiratory issues. Like peppermint, eucalyptus oil is also good with helping you to breathe a little better. Make sure if you are going to use eucalyptus oil for your allergies directly on your skin, you also use a carrier oil. Otherwise, it can be too strong and irritate your skin. Some good areas of your body to apply the diluted eucalyptus oil is on your neck, chest, and back. Inhaling it from a pot of boiling water is another way to get relief from your allergy symptoms.

Basil

When you suffer from allergies, it is not uncommon to have certain inflammatory responses to those allergens. This is often where many of your allergy symptoms come from. Basil essential oil can be helpful in reducing these responses so you are able to calm your body down. In addition to this, basil essential oil helps with killing bacteria and getting rid of mold, which also helps with your different allergy symptoms.

Some other essential oils that are good for allergies include lemon essential oil and frankincense.

Essential Oils for Anxiety

"Be aware of wonder. Live a balanced life—
learn some and think some and draw and paint and sing and dance
and play and work every day some."
~ Robert Fulgham

PEOPLE WHO suffer from anxiety or panic attacks are often looking for ways to find relief from the attacks without turning to medications. In addition to watching your diet, getting regular exercise, and finding time each day to engage in self-care, it is also a good idea to give essential oils a try. Listed below are some of the best oils for anxiety.

Lavender

Lavender is recommended for any ailment that has to do with relaxing your body since it has such a calming effect. You can relax, get better sleep, get rid of nervousness, and even reduce your overall amount of panic attacks by using lavender. Lavender is really great in a bath when you are trying to calm down, or you can put it in an oil diffuser. There are also DIY lotions and scrubs that include lavender essential oils that will also help to relax you.

Chamomile

Another relaxing and calming essential oil is chamomile. This oil helps with your anxiety, worry, and irritability. It is often recommended for people who are having trouble sleeping because it helps to relax both body and mind. However, it is not typically recommended to people with allergy problems, so if you suffer from allergies, it is a good idea to be careful.

Rose

Rose is an essential oil you can take for stress, anxiety, and depression. It is safe whether you have allergies, are pregnant or nursing, or even if you are extra sensitive to certain oils. As with all oils, just make sure your rose essential oil is properly diluted or mixed with a carrier oil. You can easily add some to a pot of boiling water and inhale it to relax or add it to a footbath to start relaxing your body.

Other Essential Oils for Anxiety

There are a lot of other essential oils you can also try for your anxiety. You can use them alone with a carrier oil or create your own blends for anxiety or stress. These oils include:

- Frankincense
- Basil
- Geranium
- Jasmine
- Clary Sage

- Lemon
- Orange
- Bergamot
- Marjoram

Try making your own blends with these essential oils to help with your anxiety. You can add some drops to a hot bath to relax your body and mind, use them in a footbath, or create your own body treatments. During a panic attack, applying oils to your skin directly with a carrier oil might give you the fastest results.

Essential Oils for Arthritis

"Find a place inside where there's joy,
and the joy will burn out the pain."

~ Joseph Campbell

IF YOU have arthritis, you know how frustrating it can be when the pain keeps you from completing normal activities. In addition to seeing your doctor for medical treatments, it is also good to try some natural remedies at home, such as with essential oils. Plants like peppermint and rosemary work very well for reducing the inflammation and swelling brought on by arthritis.

Rosemary

Rosemary oil is a soothing oil with a light floral scent that can also be used for arthritis. This is one of the top essential oils to be used for promoting better circulation. It also has anti-inflammatory benefits, so the inflammation and dwelling in your joints can be remedied with some rosemary oil. It also has anti-pain properties, which is another great reason to use it for arthritis. For arthritis, use the rosemary oil with a carrier oil like coconut oil, then rub it directly onto your joints.

Peppermint

Peppermint is an essential oil that works for so many ailments, but primarily body pain and inflammation issues. Peppermint oil, like rosemary oil, has anti-inflammatory properties. This means it is going to be tremendously helpful when reducing the inflammation that is leading to your joint pain. You might not be able to cure your arthritis, but you can bet this oil will help. You also want to use it with a carrier oil before applying to the painful joints you have. Coconut oil is a great carrier oil to use with peppermint oil.

Turmeric

You might not hear about turmeric much, but this is an herb that is really great for arthritis. Turmeric is another anti-inflammatory herb that helps, especially with rheumatoid arthritis. The herb itself is often given to people either as a supplement or to put in their food if they have arthritis. You may also want to try a turmeric tea to help with your arthritis pain.

Frankincense

Frankincense essential oil is also good for helping with ailments that are worsened by irritation and inflammation, such as with arthritis. Frankincense oil not only reduces overall inflammation, but it can also help with the breakdown of cartilage issue, reducing the severity of it.

When you are using essential oils for arthritis, applying it directly to the skin is usually the better option. As with other oils on your skin, just make sure it includes a carrier oil. However, if adding it to a bath, it is okay to skip the carrier oil.

Essential Oils for Insect and Bug Bites

"Following the basic laws of the Universe leads us to a life of total and complete joy in every moment."

~ Arnold Patent

WHEN YOU get a bug bite, it can cause stinging and burning, itching, and redness around the area where you were bit. If you use essential oils on the bite, it can help relieve many of these symptoms and speed up the healing process. Try out some of these oils for your insect or bug bites.

Lavender

Did you know lavender can be really effective with bug and insect bites as well? If you have a spot on your body that is extremely itchy and starts to burn after scratching it, it is very likely a bug bite of some kind. Keep in mind not all insect bites will make themselves known right away. When you have an itch, try mixing lavender oil with a carrier oil, such as almond or coconut oil, then apply it to the bite. Do this for all bites and itchy spots, and you should find some relief within a few days.

Eucalyptus

Eucalyptus is an essential oil that many people are surprised by. It has benefits for your physical and mental state, helping with things like anxiety and skin conditions. It also happens to be an excellent choice when you have burns, cuts and scrapes, or various types of bug bites. It will soothe the bite so that the itching and burning isn't as severe, which is really all you can ask for when you have a bug bite that is bothering you. You might also be able to apply it to your skin with a carrier oil before going outside to repel certain insects.

Tea Tree

One of the best essential oils for your skin is tea tree oil. Many people use this oil for extra moisture and to help get rid of scars. It also happens to work very well when you have a bug or insect bite. Tea tree oil is good for boosting your immune system, which can help reduce the overall effect of being bitten by certain types of bugs. In fact, it is often given to people with bites from places like Guatemala, China, Florida, and Australia. You want to make sure you use a carrier oil or dilute it with water, but it is good to bring with you on hiking or camping trips just in case you get a bite.

Many people use this oil for extra moisture and to help get rid of scars.

Basil and Thyme

Herbal essential oils like basil and thyme are both great for insect and bug bites. Basil essential oil is an anti-inflammatory oil, so it can help reduce the irritation and swelling around your bug bites. This further helps to help soothe the bite. You might also want to try using thyme essential oil, which reduces infection of your bug bite if the skin opens.

Essential Oils for Infants

*"Release the joy that is inside of another,
and you release the joy that is inside of you."*
~ Neal Donald Walsh

WHILE ESSENTIAL oils are usually reserved for adults, there are some instances where kids can also use them. You just need to be extra careful with the type you use and how you administer them to your children.

Essential Oils for Babies

First of all, you need to be really careful about what essential oils you use with your baby. You need to make sure they are diluted and that the proper carrier oil is used. If you fail to do this, your baby could become ill. There are also only certain essential oils that are good to use on babies. The oils include dill, lavender, chamomile, and blue yarrow. Make sure with chamomile, you only use German chamomile, not any other varieties.

Essential Oils for Mental Focus

"Focus on the journey, not the destination.
Joy is found not in finishing an activity but in doing it."
~ **Greg Anderson**

IF YOU have been struggling with a lack of proper mental focus and concentration, you might be looking for ways to improve it. Natural remedies are highly recommended and can be very beneficial, such as using certain types of essential oils. Take a look at these different oils that are perfect for improving mental focus and clarity.

Rosemary

Rosemary is listed as a good essential oil for many mental and emotional conditions, from high amounts of stress, to anxiety and depression. So it should come as no surprise that it is also recommended for proper mental focus. If you have issues with your memory, concentration, or focusing for long periods of time, rosemary essential oil added to your oil diffuser is a great place to start. The scent makes you concentrate better and can help alleviate the emotional stress that might be taking away from your focus.

Basil

Believe it or not, basil essential oil is often used for mental disorders, and can work very well when you want better mental focus and concentration. It has a refreshing scent that can eliminate distraction and really help with your overall memory. Whether you need it to study, get your work done, or simply have better mental focus for various projects, basil essential oil is a really good one to start with.

Cyprus

You might not hear about Cyprus essential oil much, but you should try using it for your mental focus. This oil isn't often used for physical conditions, but it can be very effective when you are experiencing problems with your concentration or focus. If you are trying to get through college, it can help you focus when studying for exams. If you are falling asleep at work or having trouble starting a new business, this will help with your concentration and overall memory.

Peppermint

A lot of the essential oils that work good with mental focus have earthy or minty scents because they don't relax you like lavender and chamomile, but instead wake up your mind. You are more alert and it works similar to caffeine in the morning. There is a spicy and minty scent to peppermint that is really great when you are waking up early and don't want to keep fueling your mind and body with caffeine from coffee or soft drinks. It can also help with headaches, so that is another bonus.

Essential Oils for Skin and Beauty

"When you wish someone joy, you wish them peace, love, prosperity, happiness—all the good things."

~ Maya Angelou

THE OIL from various plants and herbs isn't just good for your overall health, but can help with your skin and beauty as well. Take a look at some of these essential oils that will help to protect your skin from UV rays, get rid of acne and breakouts, and moisturize your skin naturally.

Ylang Ylang

When you are making your own skin or beauty products, a lot of recipes will call for ylang ylang. This is an essential oil that is great for reducing the signs of aging. It is often found in face and hand creams, and elixirs that are supposed to help to naturally remove fine lines and wrinkles. It is also great if you have acne or oily skin. It should be added to almond oil as a carrier if you are applying the essential oil directly to your skin.

Lemongrass

Another essential oil that is really good for your skin is lemongrass oil. All essential oils need to be diluted with a carrier oil if you are going to apply it to your skin, so try it with some jojoba, coconut, or grapeseed oil. Lemongrass is best for skin conditions like acne and large pores, as well as for using as a skin toner. Most store-bought skin toner products are much too harsh for your skin, but this is light and natural, so it helps with the natural skin glow that doesn't cause irritation.

Lavender

If you have skin irritation, bug bites, or burns and scrapes, try using lavender essential oil on your skin. Make sure you don't use straight essential oil on your skin since it can irritate it. Use it with a carrier oil and apply only a small amount or make your own lavender body spray that is soothing and cooling. There are a lot of recipes for making your own spritzes and sprays that use lavender to help soothe your skin and reduce the itching and soreness of burns, cuts, and scrapes.

Geranium

An essential oil not often recommended, but highly underrated, is geranium essential oil. This is good for all skin types, is soothing, and is very moisturizing. It is good for skin that is sensitive or already irritated and won't add to the irritation. If the oil balance in your skin is keeping it from a good glow and proper hydration, then geranium essential oil will be great. You can also create a face mist by adding a few drops to a spray bottle with mineral water inside.

Essential Oils for Beautiful Skin

WHILE ESSENTIAL oils are mainly used for mental health, they can also be used to help fight off painful acne. The benefits of essential oils on acne can eliminate current acne and keep your skin beautiful and healthy. Your skin is sensitive to environmental changes, stress, and oily buildup that can lead to dreadful acne. Some essential oils have the ability to fight off acne breakouts. Some people take medication to fight off acne without knowing their side effects. Using essential oils is a way to naturally remove acne and keep your skin clear.

Using essential oils is a way to naturally remove acne and keep your skin clear.

Essential oils are non-greasy, so they will not cause a buildup and clog your pores. They will do quite the contrary. In fact, using essential oils on acne is a good way to spot treat existing acne without using harsh treatments. The list below discusses several essential oils that will help you fight acne, remove blemishes, and tighten small premature wrinkles.

You may already use essential oils without your knowledge. Some manufacturers of fine creams and moisturizers already use essential oils in small amounts in their ingredient list. The fragrance can be detected in some creams that you buy over the counter. Designing your perfect beauty regimen is difficult to do without the use of essential oils. Their benefits bring healthy skin and a smooth, radiant glow to your facial features. The essential oils used in popular acne products have been used for therapeutic effects for years.

Essential oils are often dissolved in cream or oil and then applied as a moisturizer. Even in small concentrations they provide medicinal advantages over acne breakouts. The oils bring oxygen and nutrients to the skin, helping it fight off any blemishes. Below is a list of some of the most popular essential oils that will help with your acne treatments.

Clary Sage

Clary sage is extracted from plants that greatly imitate the body's own hormones. The use of clary sage is often implemented where acne stems from hormonal imbalances. The essential oil can act as a precursor allowing the body to balance its hormones.

Eucalyptus

Eucalyptus is a popular plant extract that helps your body fight off blackheads. It has a cleansing effect that removes dirt and oils and leaves only clear skin.

Lavender

Lavender is considered an all-purpose oil since its uses include acne treatment as well as mental fatigue rejuvenation. Lavender is good for the skin, and it can calm your mind and soothe your muscles from the stress and anxiety from the day.

Lemon

The citrus effects of lemon can help refresh your mind and restore your skin's natural balance. Lemon oil is known to quickly clear up current acne and remove blemishes. After applying lemon, one should be careful not to have over-exposure to the sun since it can cause skin discoloration.

Myrrh

Myrrh is a popular, ancient essential oil that was used as a balm to treat sores and scars. It can be used to treat rashes and acne breakouts. Myrrh has a variety of uses including elimination of warts or acne-causing bacteria.

Patchouly

Patchouly is a good essential oil to fight off many skin conditions. It will help you fight off acne, but it is also a good way to treat rashes and scarring. It can be used as a moisturizer as well and its fragrance will give you a calming effect.

Essential Oils for Women's Health

"I define joy as a sustained sense of well-being and internal peace—a connection to what matters."

~ Oprah Winfrey

ESSENTIAL OILS have a lot of excellent uses, and among them are some uses particularly for women. They can help with anything from your emotional state during pregnancy, to body changes each month during menstruation, all the way through menopause.

Clary Sage

Clary sage is an essential oil that contains phytoestrogens. These are really important for all things concerning women's health, but primarily when it comes to menstruation and menopause. Clary sage has a soothing scent that isn't overpowering, but does relax you with some aromatherapy properties. You might even find that clary sage essential oil can help to uplift your mood when dealing with irritability or depression during different parts of your menstrual cycle. However, if you have fibroids, you should reconsider using clary sage.

Lemon

Lemon essential oil has a crisp, fresh scent that is hard not to love. Lemon essential oil still has some of the vitamin C that lemons themselves have, which provide antioxidants for your body. These can help you to feel refreshed even on a day when you have menopause or are on your period and really don't feel your best. Try adding some essential oil to a glass of warm water or tea, or making a face cream that has lemon essential oil in it.

Lavender

Lavender essential oil is often used for many different purposes, from emotional and mental health, to insomnia and body aches and pains. It can also be great for balancing your hormones and reducing pain from menstrual cramps and other health disorders having to do with your reproductive system. If you often have headaches or stress during your period or menopause, this essential oil can help you. Lavender is also good for relieving other symptoms of PMS if you want to go the natural route. Take a nice hot bath when you have menstrual cramps and add in some drops of lavender, or add them to a diffuser when lying down.

Peppermint

If you don't mind the minty scent of peppermint, it can be really useful for women's health. It is great when you have menstrual cramps, but mostly for headaches or migraines. Many women experience some nasty headaches when they are on their period or going through menopause, and peppermint essential oil added to a diffuser while you lie down with all the lights off is a good way to find relief.

Essential Oil Blends for Autumn

WHEN THE fall season arrives, it is a great time to get out your essential oils and put them in your diffuser. It really creates the ambiance of fall and is easy to add a wonderful aromatherapy environment to your home. Try out some of these different seasonal essential oil blends.

Ultimate Fall Blend

If all you want to smell is pure fall in your essential oil diffuser, there are some different oils that you can blend together. This doesn't include a single blend, but a list of oils you can try adding together in different combinations. Remember the more drops of a certain oil, and the stronger that particular scent will be. If you want to try patchouli but not have it strong in the blend, just a few drops should be fine. Some fall-inspired essential oils to try adding include:

- Ginger
- Patchouli
- Orange
- Nutmeg

- Clove
- Cinnamon
- Lime
- Sage
- Cardamom

Chai Tea Blend

If you are a fan of spicy chai tea, you will love making an essential oil blend that smells just like your favorite tea. Think about the ingredients you will normally put into your tea to spice it up, and you can probably guess what essential oils might be used for a chai essential oil blend for the fall. Some ideas are ginger, clove, and cardamom essential oils. Make sure that when using an oil diffuser, you combine the oils with water for your blends.

Fall Citrus Blend

In the fall, many seasonal blends will also have some citrus in them. This allows you to smell the sweet scent of your favorite citrus fruits that are in season in the fall, while also enjoying the aromatherapy in your home with a diffuser. Some oils to include in a fall seasonal citrus blend include orange, lemon, cinnamon, clove, and ginger. Add your oils to some water before putting them in the diffuser. You can also try these blends in your bath for a sweet-smelling seasonal experience.

> You can also try these blends in your bath for
> a sweet-smelling seasonal experience.

Essential Oils for Energizing Yourself

*"True joy is that which gives us more energy and
makes us feel more alive."*

~ Robert Puryear

ESSENTIAL OILS can help you release stress and bring back important energy levels in your daily active life. Using essential oils in aromatherapy in your home, car, office, or any other place you spend vital amounts of time can help your energy levels increase. Just a day of use from these important oil products will have you feeling more vitalized and the reduced stress will allow you to deal with the day's pressures more calmly.

Using essential oils is an easy process.

Using essential oils is an easy process. Certain aromas will help with different illnesses, disease, stress, and energy. Choosing the right oil for your aromatherapy is important to help relieve the different adverse effects on the body. Once you choose your essential oil, you can place just a few drops into a burner, on a heater or even on your body in light amounts to continually benefit from the powerful scents. Throughout the day, using the essential oils will activate your body and mind with positive outcomes.

Stress is a powerfully negative effect on your body and inner strength. Aromatherapy can help reduce the stress, thereby increasing energy levels and counteracting the harmful processes of high levels of stress. Stress and energy counter each other and stress will eventually win as the day ages. Your body replenishes levels of energy after a good night's sleep, but stress can adversely affect sleep patterns allowing stress to ultimately win the battle. This will keep you tired and agitated during the day, which is why aromatherapy with essential oils will greatly benefit a busy lifestyle. With the continual backlash of work pressure, deadlines, and home care, your stress can take over your life. Essential oils help your mind and body fight back.

Not all essential oils are strong, pungent smells that travel long distances. Some essential oils are subtle and light. Even at low levels, your body is able to smell the scents and use them for positive benefits. They can help you relax and increase energy levels even at low levels.

Increasing energy is a major benefit of scents such as grapefruit and pine. You can use these essential oil smells separately or in combination for a fully powerful benefit. Each essential oil has a certain effect separately, and in combination the effects are powerfully synergistic.

Grapefruit

If you have ever peeled a fresh grapefruit for a healthy morning breakfast then you already know the refreshing benefits of grapefruit essential oils. The tangy fruit has an uplifting, stimulating effect from its citrus foundation. Use this type of oil to invigorate and create a feeling of refreshed energy.

Pine

Having a Christmas tree inside your home will help you realize the benefits of this aroma. Using this essential oil clears your mind and acts as a refreshing antiseptic. The aroma clears your head from the negative thoughts from the day and helps make your body feel positively revitalized.

Essential Oils to Improve Your Memory

"We are shaped by our thoughts; we become what we think. When the mind is pure, joy follows like a shadow that never leaves."
~ Buddha

OUR MEMORY is one of the most important functions that should be maintained and carefully exercised. Your memory can fade or it can be inhibited from stress, environment, or sickness. Memories can be triggered from certain events as well. Memory also should be exercised to help you increase your ability to retrieve information from long-term memory. While short-term memory only lasts a few seconds, it can still be exercised to increase its abilities.

Essential oils in aromatherapy can help you exercise your mind which will eventually increase your memory. Using essential oils in your home or office will help you concentrate on your work for the day, revitalize short-term memory, and even help your long-term memory retrieve information. Better memory will help you better understand the needs of those around you and help you listen and interact with your spouse, children, family, friends, coworkers, and customers/clients more effectively.

> **The fragrances will stimulate the part of your mind
> that helps your memory.**

If you have a poor memory, essential oils in aromatherapy can help improve your memory from only a few days of burning the scent. The fragrances will stimulate the part of your mind that helps your memory. Using essential oils in aromatherapy in the office will help you remember important dates, deal with customers better, and help you concentrate better on important documents or work. You can use the aromatherapy essential oils during the day as a preventative from becoming moody or irritable as well.

Using aromatherapy is also good for the college student. It is hard to juggle classes and homework without suffering from anxiety and low energy levels. The lost sleep from studying many hours can take a toll on your memory. Using essential oils during the college years can greatly increase your ability to concentrate, study, and remember what you have read. The oils can also help you remember lectures from professors when attending classes.

Whether it is a need to have better memory at school, work, or at home, rosemary is the perfect essential oil to increase your memory. It works almost immediately after using the aromatherapy techniques to help your mind focus and increase your memory.

Rosemary

Rosemary is a stimulating essential oil that helps you focus and maintain proper concentration to improve information retrieval. Diffusing rosemary in your home, office, or dorm room can rejuvenate tired muscles and help soothe weary feet from a hard day's work. It allows you to think clearly while studying or analyzing paperwork at work.

Using relaxing essential oils in aromatherapy for your home are also good for your memory. Using the essential oils while you are home after a hard day's work will help you relax and get a better night's sleep. A better night's sleep will help you wake up refreshed and ready to tackle the day. The relaxing essential oils help you rest the mind properly at night so that it can concentrate more efficiently during the day. Resting properly at night stimulates the brain by bringing essential nutrients during a relaxing night. The upcoming chapters on Essential Oils for a Good Night's Sleep and Essential Oils for Effective Relaxation offer suggestions on essential oils that will help you relax and ultimately increase your memory. They will help you sleep soundly, which is one of the best ways to increase your long- and short-term memory.

Even just a few days of using the essential oils in aromatherapy during your day's stressful events will help you lose the stress and continue to focus on the work or study material. Although memory can fade, the essential oils can help your memory return. Short-term memory and long-term memory will slowly return to you. You will feel sharper and full of energy.

Removing stress from your life is also an important way to help your memory return. The essential oils in aromatherapy will help remove the stress from your mind and body, which is better for your health. Try using a little rosemary the next time you feel stressed and unable to relax. You will start to feel refreshed from just a few days of aromatherapy.

Essential Oils for Irritability Relief

"The best and safest thing is to keep a balance in your life, acknowledge the great powers around us and in us. If you can do that, and live that way, you are really a wise man."

~ Euripides

IRRITABILITY CAN happen for a number of reasons, all stemming from negative energy. Irritability is an emotional issue that escalates from a bad day or from frustrations that span an even longer period of time. Some people try to hold in their anger, and perhaps they even succeed for a while, but sooner or later the emotional irritability bubbles to the top and causes even the most even-tempered person to finally release anger in the form of irritability.

Irritability stems from a number of issues that occur throughout the day. Deadlines at work, the pressure of the day's work, and any other stressful event can cause a person to suffer from irritability. Using essential oils in aromatherapy can greatly increase your body's ability to defend and fight back against the emotional negativity of irritability.

Irritability can also stem from home-related issues. Stay-at-home moms often suffer from irritability due to deadlines, taking care of their kids' every need, sleep-deprivation over a long period of time, not getting enough self-care or support, and the pressure to ensure everything in the household is perfect. Irritability can be greatly exacerbated from home-caring and child-rearing.

Essential oils in aromatherapy can help you resolve your irritability issues and they can help calm you for future work days. Even as your environment changes, essential oils will help you quell irritability from normal levels that can otherwise cause negative effects. Once you use essential oils for irritability relief, you will start to notice how your attitude changes. You may even see how people will respond to you differently once your attitude has changed to a more positive one.

Essential Oils for a Good Night's Sleep

"Happiness is not a matter of intensity but of balance and order and rhythm and harmony."

~ Thomas Merton

HAVING A fully restful night's sleep is important for your body and mind. Using essential oils through aromatherapy can help you maintain levels of peace, remove the day's stress, and help you sleep soundly for the ultimate refreshing morning.

Having a fully restful night's sleep is important for your body and mind.

Unsettled sleep will increase chances for increased stress and can ultimately hurt your immune system, making you susceptible to disease and illnesses. Essential oils used in aromatherapy can help you relax and sleep more soundly throughout the night. Having a good night's sleep is necessary to effectively recharge your body's batteries to make it the most efficient it can be for the next day. Quality sleep and rest is also beneficial to improving your mental energy and memory.

Getting six to seven hours of sleep is important for your body to replenish the energy levels that it has lost from the day's activities. However, sleeping a quality six hours of sleep is much more beneficial than sleeping a poor, restless ten hours of sleep.

Essential oils used in aromatherapy can help you fully relax to facilitate your ability to fall into a deep sleep, thereby qualifying your sleep as fully effective for your body's energy replenishment. You will notice the difference the next morning when you wake up and feel totally revitalized from the previous day. Not only will your energy feel replenished, but your mind and body will be much healthier from a quality night's sleep.

There are several essential oils that can help you have a good night's sleep. The most relaxing of all of the essential oils are bergamot, sage, and sandalwood. Although each has beneficial effects separately, combining all three has the best benefits for sleep on your mind and body.

Bergamot

Bergamot is a peel from an exotic fruit that smells like the popular citrus scent you get from other fruits. The potent citrus smell makes you feel refreshed and it calms your emotions to give you the euphoric feeling of a calm spirit. You can also blend bergamot with other oils to produce an uplifting feeling with a relaxing state that helps you sleep better.

Clary Sage

Clary sage is a popular essential oil to relax your spirit and it helps get rid of the restlessness from stress and an overactive emotional state. As with some other essential oils, it is distilled from the leaf of a plant that is known to relax you simply from its aromatic smell. It brings you a feeling of wellbeing and within twenty-four hours will make you feel like you can conquer the world.

Sandalwood

The sandalwood essential oil will soothe you so that you no longer feel as if the stress of the world is on your shoulders. It helps you ultimately relax and keeps your emotions at bay so that you can sleep throughout the night. The fragrance of sandalwood is great for the mind, which is the main factor for stressful, restless nights.

Although each of these bring a distinct benefit, as stated above, they are most beneficial used together. You can purchase the essential oils separately, but if you really want to have the most relaxing night of your life use them in combination. The combination of the oils will guarantee you a good night's sleep and give you the most refreshed feeling in the morning.

Essential Oils for Effective Relaxation

"Learning to live in the present moment is part of the path of joy."
~ ***Sarah Ban Breathnach***

RELAXATION IS an important part of a daily regimen. Most people focus on daily work schedules, exercise, home care, taking care of children, and other personal chores for daily living. Relaxation should always have a part in your day, but most people overlook the importance of relaxation and rest. Resting the mind and body helps refresh energy and brings back a balance of body strength and fortitude.

Relaxation essential oils also induce a mindful state of calm that helps you forget the day's stressful events or what daily chores are needed for the next day. Relaxation does not necessarily mean that you are required to sleep. Relaxation includes meditation and drawing your mind away from the stress and into a complete peaceful state. A total relaxation state soothes your whole body and reduces the tiring effects of stress and sleepless nights.

There are several essential oils that can help you relax in your home or in the office. Essential oils such as ylang ylang, and lavender will help you relax throughout the day without making you tired.

Both ylang ylang and lavender have their own unique effects, but when they are used together they produce a powerful aromatherapy to ultimately make you feel at peace.

Ylang Ylang

Ylang ylang is an extremely potent essential oil that is sensual and relaxing. The balancing effects from the exotic aroma leaves your whole body and spirit feeling relaxed. It is also a romantic aroma and it is perfect for date night or cuddling up with a loved one at night.

All of the above oils will help you throughout your day even if used individually. Used together and they will remove the heavy emotional effects of stress and tension. Removing the negative effects of the day can help you maintain your balance, and it is a major factor of dealing with anger management. You will find yourself more productive, and you will have a better, customer-service-friendly attitude. Use these essential oils in combination with other stress-relieving oils and you will find your whole presence to be more positive.

Essential Oils to Feel More Secure and Confident

"Wisdom is your perspective on life, your sense of balance, your understanding of how the various parts and principles apply and relate to each other."

~ Steven R. Covey

THE FOLLOWING essential oils can help you combat those helpless feelings of insecurity. You can use each of them separately for their individual benefits. Using them in combination creates a powerful solution for the depression and anxiety issues that contribute to insecurities. Frankincense is a great essential oil to help you prevent depression and fight off insecurities. Jasmine and lavender are two essential oils that will successfully boost your mood and help you balance your emotions. The essential oils listed below can be used separately for their individual benefits to help eliminate depression. Use them together as potent solutions to help rid yourself from depression quickly and efficiently.

Frankincense

Frankincense is a rejuvenating essential oil that will make you feel refreshed and balanced almost immediately. It is an exotic fragrance that is extracted from special bushes that are native to Africa. It has been used for thousands of years as a relaxing fragrance included as part of religious ceremonies. It is also used as an essential oil that aids in meditation. While relaxing, it also aids in uplifting and improving your mood.

Jasmine

Jasmine is a sensual essential oil that helps you assert yourself. It can relax you beyond the stressful day and it can lift your emotions. It can also boost your confidence and your self- esteem to help overcome the controversy from the day.

Lavender

Lavender is a soothing essential oil that can help you mentally relax. It is an herb from France that has become popular for its therapeutic uses. It can help balance your mood and release the tension from your mind and your muscles. It has been mentioned a few times for its various properties.

CONCLUSION

In conclusion I just want to state that God's medicine is growing all over the planet to assist people and animals alike to experience the benefits of Aroma and Therapeutic healing. I hope some of this information will spark a desire for you to experience the Young Living Oils available to all. As Christopher stated at the beginning of his journey, he is enjoying both the 20% discount he receives from signing up as a distributor and the health benefits that are provided to all Young Living Oil members. I have friends and family using the oils and we are all loving the ability to cook, clean, smell, diffuse and feel the healing benefits of the oils. You may contact any of the people listed at the beginning of this information to purchase, ask questions or set up a gathering of friends and/or relatives for a shared demonstration of the many uses of Young Living Oils. You may also join to gain the 20% discount by contacting myself or anyone in my downline.

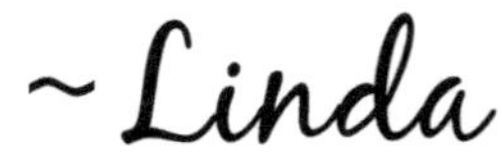